Who cares.

INFORMATION AND

SUPPORT FOR THE CARERS

OF CONFUSED PEOPLE

ACKNOWLEDGEMENTS

Original edition researched and written by Maggie Jee and Liz Reason. With grateful thanks to the steering committee and the carers' support groups, whose experience and advice form the basis of this booklet. This edition has been developed with the valuable assistance of Help the Aged, Age Concern (England) and the Alzheimer's Society to whom Health Promotion England extends its grateful thanks.

Whilst every effort has been made to ensure that details in this publication are up to date, changes in the benefits system and in social services mean that some facts may be incorrect. You are advised to check either with your local Citizens Advice Bureau or one of the other agencies listed on p.76.

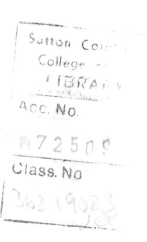

CONTENTS

INTRODUCTION

If you are reading this booklet because some of the comments on the cover struck a chord with you, you may be looking after someone who has dementia.

This booklet has been written to tell you:
- more about dementia
- what it is like for someone at home
- how to ease the problems of day-to-day care, and
- about the help available to carers.

Dementia is a distressing condition and a lot of what follows in this booklet may be painful to you. But the booklet is not primarily about dementia. It is designed to support you, the carer. It has been written with the advice of many people who are or have been carers themselves and who have shared their experiences to help others. All the examples and quotes used in the booklet are based on what different carers have said. After reading the booklet, you may want to discuss what you have read with your doctor or with a counsellor who is familiar with the condition.

It is hoped that these carers' experiences will support you in a task that may at times seem daunting and thankless and help you realise that you are not alone. Wherever possible the booklet is optimistic – not because everything will be easy, it won't – but because many carers have stressed that whatever the difficulties, there are also small triumphs to be won.

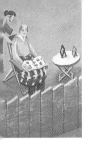

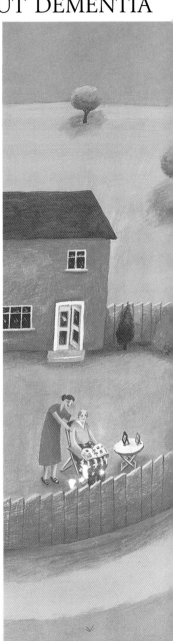

Dementia is a complex and perplexing condition. It includes a number of different diseases, of which Alzheimer's disease is the most common. As a carer you need good information and support to help you understand the condition and its consequences.

WHAT IS DEMENTIA?

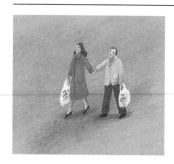

Dementia is a condition in which the cells of the brain die more quickly than in normal ageing. This leads to a general decline in a person's abilities. It can produce loss of memory, confusion, odd behaviour and personality changes. The causes are not yet understood. There is no cure for dementia, and little treatment can be offered, although new drugs are beginning to be developed that alleviate some of the symptoms of Alzheimer's disease. Since the same symptoms may result from other disorders, which may be curable, it is important to get a proper diagnosis. Dementia by itself is not usually a cause of death and someone may have the condition for several years before dying from something else.

There are two main types of dementia. Their symptoms and effects are much the same although they progress differently.

- In Alzheimer's disease changes take place in the structure of the brain, leading to cell death. The onset of the disease is gradual and the decline usually slow and regular.

- The second main type of dementia happens when 'mini' strokes take place in the brain which destroy small areas of cells. This is called 'multi-infarct' (or sometimes vascular) dementia. It often progresses in a step-like way and the onset may be sudden.

The person may not get any worse for periods of time, and may even seem to improve, although decline will be the eventual outcome. Some people have both Alzheimer's disease and multi-infarct dementia together.

Other types of dementia include Lewy body disease, Pick's disease, Parkinson's disease, Huntington's disease and Creutzfeldt-Jakob Disease (CJD).

WHO WILL GET DEMENTIA?

Dementia is usually a disease of old age, with six in a hundred people over the age of 65 developing it to some degree, increasing to twenty in a hundred among people over 85. However, it is estimated that as many as 17,000 people under the age of 65 have dementia and hence have particular and specific needs that are not necessarily dealt with in this book. Please contact the Alzheimer's Society for more information.

As far as is known, dementia occurs equally across all groups in society. Unlike many other diseases it does not appear to be linked with social class, ethnic group or geographical location.

WHAT CAUSES DEMENTIA?

Because dementia is such a distressing illness and is not fully understood you may have anxieties about the nature of the disease, especially about its causes and your own chances of getting it.

One carer admitted:
'My mother's got it, so I can't help wondering about myself. Every morning when I wake up, I think to myself, "Now what did I have last night for my meal? What day is it? Right! I haven't got it – yet!"'

But dementia is not thought to be inherited in most cases.

Many people are fearful of 'going mad' in old age, especially as mental illness is often considered to be embarrassing or shameful. Although dementia becomes more common with increasing age, this does not mean that it should be seen as part of normal ageing, nor is it caused by old age.

You may try to explain the disease by finding a 'cause' in an accident or loss which occurred about the same time as the symptoms appeared. Although its onset may coincide with major life changes such as the death of a spouse or moving house, it will not have been *caused* by it.

Nor is there any evidence to support other commonly held beliefs about the causes of dementia. It is NOT infectious and cannot be caught or sexually transmitted although some people with AIDS do develop dementia. It is NOT caused by 'over-use' or 'under-use' of the brain.

At the moment it is easier to say what does not cause dementia rather than what does. However, research into causes and treatments continues. You and the person suffering from dementia may be asked to co-operate in this research. The more people who agree, the more likely it is that a cure will be found. Regarding Alzheimer's disease itself, it is now widely accepted that when the cause is discovered, it will turn out to be a multiplicity of factors which differ from one individual to another in their ability to influence the development of the disease. These influences may involve genetic aspects, and environmental factors. The causes of other forms of dementia, such as multi-infarct dementia, CJD and Korsakoff's syndrome are now more clearly understood.

WHAT ARE THE SYMPTOMS OF DEMENTIA?

A major symptom of dementia is that the person consistently forgets things they have just said or done, although their memory for past events may remain perfectly clear. Loss of short term memory is always a feature of dementia, although it may not become noticeable for some time after the onset of the disease.

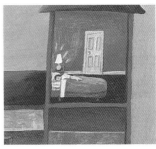

There are many other symptoms of dementia although it is unlikely that one person will develop all of them. Each person with dementia will be affected in a different way. The overall impact of the disease depends partly on what the person was like in the first place – their personality and their physical condition – and on the type of dementia they have. Some individuals become disagreeable and more difficult to live with. Others become docile and even-tempered. Some will become severely disabled while others will be able to manage for themselves with only minimum help for a long time.

Although the symptoms do not follow a regular pattern in every case, some changes are more likely to occur

The person may be forgetful, and confused:

'We were staying in a hotel we'd been to many times and he didn't seem to know his way about. He couldn't remember where the toilet was.'

Behaviour may be slightly odd or inappropriate:

He kept saying he'd lost his coat and spent ages looking for it, and he had it on all the time!' 'He bought a TV stamp and seemed very proud of himself. But it's something we never do, we never buy TV stamps.'

For others the symptoms may be more unusual:

'It started with hallucinations. He used to talk about a woman in white.'

at the onset of the disease and others as the disease progresses.

This booklet starts with those changes most common in early dementia – changes which may well be unrecognised at the time and only fit into a pattern of declining ability when the carer looks back. It then describes the symptoms that may develop during the course of dementia. Finally, the booklet gives you an idea of the most severe problems you may have to face, even though this may be worrying and painful if you are at the beginning of caring.

In the early stages of the disease an often-mentioned change is that the person seems different from their usual self in ways that may be hard to pin-point. Their approach to life is dulled, they seem less capable, less involved and less adaptable in all spheres of life. They may show loss of concentration, seem unable to make decisions or avoid taking responsibility. Carers have described the person as 'not the man he was' or as if 'the life had gone out of her' or as having 'lost her brightness'. More tangible changes may accompany this dullness.

The person with dementia may be just as puzzled by their own behaviour. They may become upset and irritated by their own incompetence, or more wrapped up in themselves. These mood changes may be noticeable to family and friends too but not necessarily seen as causes for alarm. And at this stage of the disease it is still possible to make excuses or allowances for these changes – to put them down to overwork, worry and so on.

As the disease progresses the symptoms become more obvious and disabling. Individuals may:

- be very forgetful, especially of recent events and people's names
- be muddled about time, day, place, and unable to find their way around familiar surroundings
- have difficulty in talking, and often repeat themselves
- be unable to make sense of what is said to them
- have difficulty carrying out household tasks and neglect personal hygiene
- put themselves at risk by leaving pans to boil dry or gas fires unlit
- behave inappropriately, like going out in their nightclothes or wandering around the streets at night
- hide or lose things and accuse others of stealing them
- see or hear things that are not there
- become angry, upset or aggressive very easily.

In the final stages of the disease people may:

- be unable to remember things they have just said or done
- not recognise known faces and familiar objects
- be unable to express themselves
- be unable to understand what is said to them
- be very restless, especially at night

The following examples, recorded by carers, are typical:

'After a couple of years she couldn't put a name to things.'

'I spoke to him about a plug that wasn't working and all I got was gibberish.'

'He stayed in the bedroom one and a half hours to tie his tie...oh! the frustration!...He couldn't tie his shoe-laces either, the laces would be at the side, and he'd put his underwear on back to front.'

'She could see two men at the end of the bed and swarms of animals crawling over the wardrobe.'

- try to carry out actions or relive events from their past
- be unable to carry out household and personal hygiene tasks without a lot of help and supervision
- have bladder and bowel incontinence
- have to use a wheelchair
- be bedridden.

WHY SHOULD YOU GET A DIAGNOSIS?

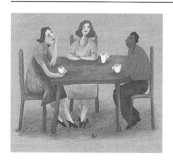

It is very important to get a proper medical diagnosis if a middle aged or older person develops some of these symptoms and does not get any better. This is because many other conditions which may be treatable can give rise to some of the symptoms of dementia and might be mistaken for it.

For example, memory loss and confusion are symptoms of incurable dementia, but could also be due to other causes especially if they arise suddenly.

These are the more usual things which cause dementia-like symptoms:

- Almost any infection of the body such as pneumonia or kidney infection. Treatment of the infection will cure the symptoms.
- Thyroid gland deficiency or vitamin deficiency which may be completely cured.
- Chemical deficiency, as in Parkinson's disease, which can be controlled.
- Other brain disorders. Brain tumours, strokes or head injuries may temporarily or permanently affect

parts of the brain, leading to confusion and other symptoms of dementia. These conditions can sometimes be treated and cured.

- Almost any drug. Older people generally do not need such large doses of drugs as younger people. Even the effects of common drugs such as sleeping tablets last much longer in an older person. They may also be taking several drugs which in combination could produce dementia-like symptoms. When the dosage is corrected the symptoms disappear.
- Severe depression. It is common in older people and usually treatable.
- Changes in the person's relationships such as the serious illness or death of a spouse or close friend.
- Changes in the person's usual habits or environment such as moving house.

It is difficult to make a conclusive diagnosis of dementia but tests can eliminate most of these other causes of the symptoms. Usually, if no other reason can be found for the symptoms, dementia will be diagnosed. Although it is hard to accept a diagnosis of incurable dementia most carers agree that it is best to know the truth so that people can plan for their friends and family and think about what they would like in future. It is also easier to accept that someone is *ill* rather than just 'odd' or 'difficult'. When people remain undiagnosed for several years, or if the process of diagnosis is very prolonged, they and their carers generally suffer increased anxiety and frustration.

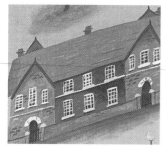

Even if the person is found to have incurable dementia some of their *symptoms* may be treatable. Sometimes, dementia is accompanied by other conditions which may worsen. Often these can be treated.

If you are looking after someone with dementia-like symptoms, ask your doctor to start the process of diagnosis (see *Medical help* on p.36.) When, and only when, a diagnosis of dementia has been made, there will be some difficult decisions to be reached (see the next section *Your emotions as a carer* and *General guidelines for caring* on p.41.)

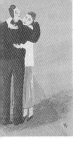

YOUR EMOTIONS AS A CARER

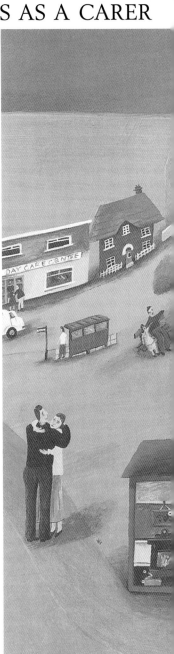

P eople find themselves looking after a confused person at home for many different reasons – out of love, from a sense of duty, perhaps because they feel they have no choice. Some find assuming the responsibility relatively easy. Others come increasingly to resent it. This chapter suggests ways of coping and coming to terms with your emotions.

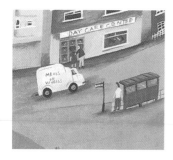

However you approach your caring responsibilities they will certainly arouse a great many conflicting emotions in you, and in your family. In part, your response will be affected by your relationship with the individual. Spouses caring for partners will almost certainly experience different feelings from sons or daughters caring for parents, or a sister for a brother. And whether the previous relationship between the individual and carer has been close or distant, whether there has been love and companionship or indifference and dislike will affect the strength and range of your emotions.

So many of these emotions are negative that it is easy to become overwhelmed by them, and to feel that you are alone in trying to cope with them. But you are not alone. All these emotions – and no doubt others besides – have been experienced by carers other than yourself and are a common part of the caring process. Finding other carers to talk to as soon as you can should help you to come to terms with your feelings and provide much needed support (see *Help for the carer* on p.23.)

While you may feel any or all of these emotions at any time, certain feelings may occur at different stages, usually linked to the progress of the disease or to your understanding of it.

IN THE BEGINNING

You will have noticed some of the symptoms before you know the person is ill, probably before you have had any professional advice or outside help from any source. You are likely to be puzzled, bewildered, even alarmed. What accounts for the odd and upsetting changes in behaviour and personality? You will probably be trying to find an explanation on the one hand – 'he's working too hard' – and denying that there is a problem on the other – 'After all, she's always been a bit absent-minded.' But inside, you may be afraid because you sense an almost indescribable change which you don't understand. Other people may not have noticed anything amiss. Even your doctor may dismiss your fears lightly. For many carers this may be a very difficult time – and the time when least help and support will be available or offered.

'Why is he behaving like this?'

'What's the matter with her?'

'I must be imagining things.'

WHEN THE ILLNESS IS DIAGNOSED

Not that it's easy once a diagnosis has been made. It may be reassuring to have it confirmed that the person really is ill – and you can begin to prepare for the changes that will have to take place in your lives. But it will take a while for the implications of the disease to sink in. It may be hard, if not impossible to accept that there is no cure and that the person will not get better. You will be apprehensive about how you will manage in the future and anxious about whether the sick person will suffer. You may be overwhelmed by the prospect of having to care for someone who may become very ill and angry that fate has singled you out.

'Why can nothing be done?'

'Is she really not going to get better?'

'Why me? Why us?'

'I hated everybody at first. I had a grudge against everything and everybody.'

'I shall never come to terms with it as long as I live.'

There are no glib assurances for any of these misgivings and carers differ in their ability to come to terms with the diagnosis.

'At the beginning you think you will never cope, but if you love a person and you're with them all the while, you do. It's hard, it's very, very hard, but you do grow into it, you learn by your mistakes.'

Carers do not find their task easy. But many agree that there is a process of becoming a carer which can be learned, and which makes caring less of a burden.

Caring can also bring its own rewards – satisfaction when things go well, an opportunity to express your love for the sufferer, or perhaps to return care that you received as a child.

COPING WITH CARING

'Why don't other people understand?'

'How will I cope?'

'Is this still the man I was married to for 40 years?'

By this stage, the illness may be causing real difficulties in carrying out normal day-to-day activities, and this will be the time when you may have to make major adjustments to your way of life. Ordinary tasks like dressing and eating a meal may take twice or three times as long as they used to. Some very irritating ways of behaving may have developed and the illness may be straining family relationships. Teenage children may find it particularly difficult to adjust. Such problems are likely to make you feel tense and anxious until you find ways of getting round some of them.

You may feel hurt by changes in the individual's personality and their responses to you. An affectionate gesture may not be returned or even recognised.

Nevertheless, you may feel very protective towards them, and caring for them can bring strong feelings of tenderness and compassion.

The illness may also become more obvious to outsiders, and some of the things the person does may cause you severe embarrassment, especially when strangers, or even friends, don't understand or are intolerant of odd behaviour. Because of such difficulties, you may find that you become isolated from your former social life, and that you are feeling increasingly lonely. You should do your best to avoid this. (*Personal support for the carer* on p. 37 suggests ways of avoiding it.) Anyway, you don't always owe people an explanation, but you may be pleasantly surprised about how well they react once they understand the situation.

But, however well you adapt to the new situation, feelings of anger and aggression are certain to surface from time to time. You may feel angry that this has happened to you. You may be frustrated that more is not known about the disease so that effective treatment and a cure can be offered. Doctors and other professionals may seem unconcerned and slow to provide help, as may other members of your family. And at times you will get angry with the person and their irritating behaviour.

Sometimes carers reach a point where they are physically aggressive towards the individual. This is a clear signal that the carer needs a break from the situation and more support. This can be obtained from

'I told some of the old ladies round here. I told them "Now Clifford's getting forgetful he may do odd things, he may come and knock at your door." One old lady said "By Jove, I'd be glad if he did. I've not had a man to see me for ages!"'

'That Saturday he followed me all over, even going to the toilet … it really got me uptight. I told him to get away from me but he didn't. I had to beg him to get away. He went out of the kitchen and I slammed the door after him.'

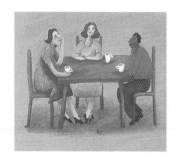

social services, Age Concern and the Carer's National Association. There is also the Elder Abuse Response Line 080 8808 8141 which is available from 10 a.m. – 4.30 p.m. Mon – Fri for those who are concerned about abusing the person they are caring for.

Losing your temper with the individual is something that carers often feel guilty about, although it may be reassuring to know that most carers admit to it. People also feel guilty about many other things – for the way they treated the sufferer in the past, for resenting having to look after them, for wanting them to go into permanent care, or for wishing them to die. Feeling guilty is a common and understandable reaction when confronted with a trying and often inexplicable disease like dementia, though feeling guilty will probably do neither you nor the individual much good. One carer confessed that he had sometimes had trouble coping but he saw no reason why he should feel guilty about being less than perfect (see left).

'I've heard the word "guilt" used...it gets up my nose. I don't feel guilt at all and I think it's an abomination that people should use the word guilt when a carer has been looking after someone as best they can...'

Indeed carers ought to feel pride at what they have done in difficult circumstances rather than guilt for what they have not managed to do.

You may also feel frightened if you have to take over making decisions in the family which were previously made by the person concerned. Remember that specialists have told you that their patient can no longer manage their own life. If you don't accept the

20

responsibility, things will not run smoothly for either of you. When you have to do it, it is reassuring how much you can accomplish, with the right support and help.

IN THE FINAL STAGES

The individual's personality may have changed almost beyond recognition, and they may have lost many of their faculties. This is certainly more distressing for the carer, who is keenly aware of what is happening, than it may be for the person themself.

You may at this time experience a great sense of sadness and may begin to mourn the loss of the person you once knew. You may also find that you can no longer cope with the situation and reach a state of despair. You may wonder what all the hard work and emotionally exhausting care is for and ask yourself: 'What's the point – wouldn't she be better off dead?'

If this happens, you should look at alternatives. Caring at home does not necessarily have to last until the death of the person in your care. If the stress of caring becomes too great, you should definitely consider giving up your responsibility and having the individual looked after permanently in residential or nursing care. This does not mean, of course, that you will cease to care. Carers emphasise the benefits of visiting the individual in their new home and say that it can restore a relationship that has been soured by the stresses of caring.

'To think of him, bless his heart, he's always been a good son and a wonderful husband...to have this degrading business happen to him. One thing I will say – he doesn't know – which is fortunate.'

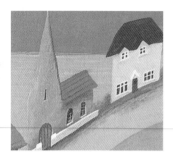

The transfer to permanent care in a home may induce a sense of grief, almost as if the sufferer had already died: 'When she first went in, I can only say it was like a bereavement.' But visiting regularly can be important, even if the person doesn't recognise you: 'It's a form of therapy for you – the figure of the person, although the character's gone.'

For some, this period of grieving before death will mean that you have begun the mourning process and started saying your goodbyes. This is a natural reaction to the prolonged stresses of caring without receiving a response from the person concerned. You should not let other people's opinions upset you if they do not understand your reaction. It is quite a usual one.

After the person's death you may at first feel a great relief that so much suffering is over. It could be some while before the normal process of bereavement takes place. You may also have to grieve twice over – once for the person with the dementia and once for the person you knew and loved before their illness.

If you have been caring for a long time and have given up your job and much of your social life you may need help to pick up the pieces and start again. Contact the Carers National Association which sometimes runs ex-carers' groups at a local level.

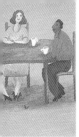

HELP FOR THE CARER

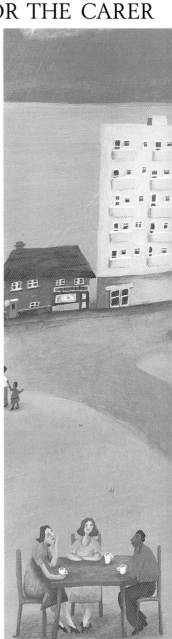

Looking after someone with dementia at home can be distressing, and is almost always hard work. But many carers say that they also get satisfaction from helping the person, and still have some good times together. Certainly many carers want to keep their relatives at home until caring becomes too heavy a burden. But if you are going to care for someone with dementia at home, it is essential that you should seek help.

WHY SHOULD YOU SEEK HELP?

It is important to realise that coping at home can cause severe strain to you, the carer. You may be elderly yourself, not in the best of health, and have difficulty with the physical demands of caring. If the person lives alone in their own home, you will have the responsibility of running two households and the worry of wondering what is happening when you're not there. You may even have to spend a lot of your caring time travelling between your home and theirs. Having the person live with you and your family may cause tensions because of the demands they make on the household.

Whatever the arrangement, caring for someone with dementia is likely to have effects on your health, family life, leisure and finances. That is why you should always seek help as soon as you suspect that your relative is ill. Don't wait until you're desperate before you ask for help. An extra pair of hands, some time off for you to relax, or a bit of extra income may be enough to see you through a crisis.

Even if you don't think you need help now, find out what is available and how long it takes to arrange – in some cases it may be weeks or even months. Then when you sense you're going to need help, you can try and start the process in good time.

Always be prepared to ask for help. Services are provided because it is known they are needed by people like you, and it is your right to ask for them. And don't forget, *your* well-being is as important as that of the person with dementia.

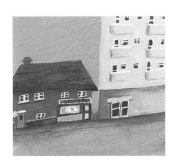

There are four main areas of help you should know about – medical, personal, practical and financial. Key addresses are provided in *Useful organisations* on p.76.

Medical help

Your doctor is the first person you should contact when you suspect that your relative is ill so that you can get a proper diagnosis of their illness. Doctors vary greatly in their attitudes towards dementia patients. Some aren't interested, some are inexperienced or not very knowledgeable about the condition, others may wish to protect you from knowing the worst about the disease and so appear to be unconcerned. Others are very helpful, being both sympathetic and providing practical help.

Carers have suggested that you need to be firm and persistent with doctors who aren't immediately helpful. If you are really getting nowhere it is legally possible to change your doctor, although this is not always practically possible. If you wish to change your doctor, you can simply go to a new doctor – or visit several and then choose – and then ask to be put on the list. If the new doctor agrees, then the

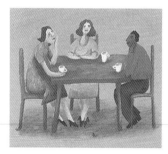

arrangements will be made through the new doctor and the health authority. If you can't find a doctor, then the health authority must assist.

Doctors must now arrange an annual check up for everyone aged over 75. You may want to make sure that you can be present at this check up. At the check up, which can be done in the person's home, there should be a chance to talk about problems which the person with dementia has.

A good doctor will act as a key to all the other services provided by the National Health Service. This will include referral to hospital specialists for further diagnosis if necessary, and for treatment. A doctor can also provide access to community nursing staff who can help and advise you at home. Normally, your doctor is the only person who can refer you to hospital specialists unless a patient is admitted for emergency treatment. Hospital specialists can also put you in touch with community nursing staff.

You should also make full use of your local social services office, voluntary organisations and carers and support groups. You can contact all of these directly: see p.76.

Are there any drugs or medication that might help? Sadly, there are very few but two drugs, Aricept and Exelon, have now been licensed in the UK specifically to treat Alzheimer's disease. However, they are not a cure for the disease, nor do they appear to stop or slow down its progression, although they do stop or slow down the development of symptoms of many people with the disease. For more information contact the Alzheimer's Society (see p.76). Sometimes, medication to calm someone is useful, but it is important to use the correct dose as some individuals can be very sensitive to these drugs. Of course it's also very important to treat other illnesses, like bronchitis, quickly and you should see your doctor if there is a sudden, if minor, change.

Personal support for the carer

A major risk for carers is that you may become socially isolated. Looking after someone with dementia takes more and more of your time. Their odd behaviour may annoy or embarrass friends and neighbours who may stop calling round. You may become afraid to leave them alone at home because they have become a danger to themselves. But struggling to manage on your own increases the stress on you, and reduces your ability to cope. Stopping yourself from becoming isolated is an essential part of coping with caring.

There are three main things you can do:

- First, make sure that you get a break from caring – some time to pursue your own interests or hobbies, to visit friends, or simply to get on with everyday tasks without having to worry about supervising the other person. The break may be for just one evening

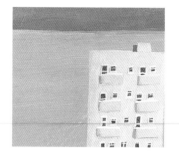

a week, for one or several days a week, or even time for a proper holiday. However long, the idea is to give you a rest or the opportunity to continue your job. Getting a break may also help the individual, offering them a chance to socialise with others and take part in different stimulating activities. Many carers find day-care useful and suggest that you start it as soon as possible so that the day-care staff can learn to adapt to any problems as they worsen. Your doctor or local social services department should be able to help you arrange a break.

- Second, carers can never stress enough the benefits of talking to other people who understand your problems. Those most able to understand are obviously other carers. Carers' support groups, where carers meet regularly to share their experiences and to help each other, exist in many parts of the country. Where no group already exists, you might want to set one up yourself. The Alzheimer's Society or the Carers' National Association, listed under *Useful organisations* on p.76, will be able to help and advise you.

- Third, where at all possible, you should try to share the responsibility for caring with other members of your family, or with friends and neighbours. Women, in particular, often find that they are expected to care for a sick relative though many carers are, in fact, men. Both women and men carers should encourage others to help them. Family members may not realise how hard a time you're having unless you tell them. Until you ask for help they may assume you don't need it. Sharing housework and organising care rotas would spread the load more fairly. Friends and neighbours may be able to help in many ways, particularly if you explain the illness, and its effects on the sufferer and on you.

Practical help
The medical and social services and some voluntary organisations may be able to offer help with a number of practical tasks in the home, such as providing regular nursing care, home helps and meals-on-wheels. They may also supply safety aids for the bathroom or stairs, equipment such as commodes, and a laundry service. If you can afford it, it is worth spending money on anything that will relieve you of daily tasks, such as a washing machine.

If you are sure that you have made full use of all possible help available at home but you are starting to find it increasingly difficult to cope, you should find out whether it will be possible to have the person with dementia cared for permanently in a residential or nursing home. The availability of such care varies throughout the country, and the ways of paying for it are complex. It is very important that you seek good advice about what kind of care may be possible: contact one of the useful organisations on p.76.

The following is just a brief description of how care might be arranged.

If you feel you will need help with paying for residential care you should contact your local social services office. They will also advise more generally on the availability of residential and nursing homes in your area. Useful organisations are the Elderly Accommodation Counsel and Counsel and Care, see pp.76–7. Help the Aged publish a leaflet, *Residential care.*

Your choice of private care also depends on what you can afford, although there is state help in many cases. You should obtain a proper diagnosis of the sufferer's illness before they go into private care. You may have to be very persistent to obtain permanent care, so don't give up hope if you fail at the first, second or even third attempt.

Financial help

Finally, caring may substantially alter your financial circumstances. You may have to go part-time or give up your job altogether; fuel bills may rise because more time at home means more heating; laundry costs and money spent on clothing may increase if the sufferer becomes incontinent.

Both you and the person you care for may be entitled to extra cash in the form of welfare or disability benefits. To find out what you may be entitled to, contact your local Benefits Agency (Social Security) office. You will find their phone number and address in the phone book under Social Security or Benefits Agency. You can also get leaflet SD1 *Sick or disabled?* from your Social Security office or post office.

You can also ring the Benefit Enquiry Line for people with disabilities (0800 88 22 00) – a freephone number which can give confidential advice to people with disabilities and their carers. Open Monday to Friday, 8.30 a.m. – 6.30 p.m., Saturday 9.00 a.m. – 1.00 p.m. Advisers can even go through a claim form over the phone and fill it in for you. If you want, they will send you information in a letter after your call. They can also provide leaflets giving more details. Information on more specific benefits is given on pp.39–40. The Benefits Agency's leaflet, *Caring for someone?* (SD4) is aimed specifically at carers. Website: www.dss.gov.uk

Don't give up
The medical, practical and carer support services will vary according to where you live. Some areas are well provided with services, others less so. You should find out now what is available near you, and keep a record of how and where to make contact. There is space to do this on the back cover of this booklet. Go to your local social services office and ask for an assessment for the services that are available – both for yourself and the one you care for. Look under your Local Authority in the telephone directory. Alternatively, your

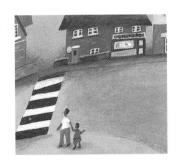

doctor may be able to help. The library and Citizens Advice Bureau will also be able to help, and the *Useful organisations* section at the back of this booklet will give you some ideas too. Remember it is your right to ask for the medical and social services that are available in your area, and you need to take up what is on offer before a difficult task becomes impossible and leads to your own ill health.

'We'd been trying to persuade our doctor to do something for months. Finally he contacted a specialist. We didn't know anything about it – until the specialist just called on mother at home. And he's been wonderful ever since, putting us in touch with so much other help.'

Many carers become extremely discouraged if several attempts to get help have failed. But it is worth persevering. Most carers eventually find their way into the network and are relieved and even delighted by the help that is provided.

As always, the first step is the hardest. The support you get will be worth your extra effort.

A WHO'S WHO OF HELP

Your local health authority
- your doctor can refer you to the following hospital and community services.

Hospital services
- a psychiatrist – specialist in mental illness for any age group
- a neurologist – specialist in diseases of the brain and nervous system
- a geriatrician – specialist in diseases of the elderly
- a clinical psychologist – specialist in mental and behavioural functions of the brain

- a psycho-geriatrician (or old age psychiatrist) – specialist in mental illness among the elderly.

Community services
- a district nurse provides nursing care at home
- a health visitor provides general health advice at home (you can ask to see one for yourself at your local health centre or clinic)
- a community psychiatric nurse provides nursing care for mentally ill people at home. Sometimes there are aids for practical care
- a continence adviser offers advice about the management of incontinence
- a chiropodist provides foot care
- an annual health check must be offered by the general practice every year to look at needs of patients over 75.

Social services
One of the first things you need to do is to get an assessment of need carried out by your local social services office. Section 2 of the 1970 Chronically Sick and Disabled Person's Act lists the services which social services have to consider during an assessment. These include day care and home help. Once social services have decided that someone needs any of the services listed in this act, they have a duty to ensure that need is met. Should the service not be available locally, then it is the ultimate responsibility of social services to ensure that the need is met by bringing in services from outside of their area.

Talk to your local social services office or hospital social worker about the assessment procedures in your area. The Carers (Recognition and Services) Act 1995 places a duty on local authorities to assess, on request, carers who provide a substantial amount of care on a regular basis. The person (or people) carrying out the assessment will look at the needs of the person with dementia *and* the carer and, in co-operation with them, try to work out the most suitable package of services. There will be an assessment of ability to pay for many of these services, and the assessor will want to ensure that all available state benefits are being claimed.

Different people may be involved in the assessment. An occupational therapist may advise on dealing with practical problems, and perhaps arrange for equipment to be provided in the home. As a result of the needs assessment, a variety of help may be arranged – meals, home care, respite breaks, day-care – depending on what is available locally. If the kind of help which you need is not available, you may need to work hard to have it arranged. This is sometimes easier to do in co-operation with others in the same situation.

VOLUNTARY ORGANISATIONS

These are charities and other non-statutory bodies, who provide many services to supplement those provided by the health and social services. There are far too many to list here, and they vary from area to area, but here are some examples:

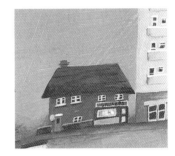

Local information and financial advice
Your nearest Citizens Advice Bureau

Carers' support groups
Age Concern*
The Alzheimer's Society (specialises in dementia*)
Mind*
Carers National Association*

Getting a break
British Red Cross Society
Age Concern*
Women's Royal Voluntary Service (WRVS)
Crossroads*

For information on schemes local to your area, contact your town hall or Citizens Advice Bureau.

*address given on pp. 76 – 7

PROBLEMS AND WHO CAN HELP

Medical help for someone with dementia

1. Finding out what's wrong

diagnosis of the illness	your doctor should refer you to a hospital specialist for an assessment

2. Regular health care

to keep a check on the progress of the illness and any other minor complaints that might be treatable.	district nurse

3. Nursing care at home

help with bathing, getting out of bed, dressing sores etc.	health visitor, district nurse
general health advice e.g. about diet, constipation	health visitor, dietitian
help with emotional and behavioural problems	community psychiatric nurse
assessment for aids such as a commode or walking frame	occupational therapist (social services or health)
difficulty in walking caused by lack of foot care	chiropodist

Your doctor or specialist should put you in touch with most of these people. You can contact the health visitor directly at your local health centre or clinic and you can contact the occupational therapy department through social services.

Personal support for the carer

1. Getting a break

sitters, minders, care attendants come into your home for a few hours a day to give you the chance to get out

social services, voluntary organisations

day care where the person with dementia is taken to a local day centre for an agreed number of days a week allowing you to go to work or have some time at home alone

social services, local health authority, voluntary organisations

short-term residential care (sometimes called respite care) where the individual goes to a home or hospital for a period of between a weekend and a month, possibly on a regular basis

social services, local health authority, voluntary organisations

permanent residential care where the individual goes into a home

social services, local health authority, voluntary organisations, private nursing or rest homes

2. Carers' emotional problems

someone to talk to

social workers, doctors, health visitors and other health workers may be sympathetic listeners

Some voluntary organisations provide trained counsellors. There is a growing network of carers' groups set up by voluntary organisations and some health authorities and social services departments. The Carers National Association and Alzheimer's Society provide excellent support in this area

You may find religion a comfort

Practical help

1. Help in the home

home care to assist with personal care, practical help around the house and shopping	social services
community meals or meals-on-wheels will provide one hot meal for an agreed number of days a week, usually only for the housebound	social services, voluntary organisations, WRVS

2. Safety

a brief demonstration of the correct method of lifting or moving the patient could avoid injury to both of you	district nurse or physiotherapist
bath aids – grab handles for the side of the bath, bath seat, bath mat, non-slip mat for inside bath, shower fitment hand rails for stairs and more major adaptations to your home such as installing a hoist or a downstairs toilet	occupational therapist for larger items; other items from bathroom shops, department stores, etc.
adaptations for cookers and fires	local electricity and gas boards, social services

3. Incontinence

treatment/management	doctor, continence adviser
incontinence pads	district nurse, continence adviser of local health authority, chemist shop
commodes	voluntary organisations, local health authorities
special clothing for protection or to make dressing and undressing easier	district nurse who can also tell you where you can buy them
laundry services, where available, may provide and wash bed linen	social services, local health authority

Financial help

You should get independent advice from your local Citizens Advice Bureau on what and how to claim *before* you go to the relevant office. Help the Aged produce two free advice leaflets *Can you claim it?* and *Claiming Disability Benefits* which provide excellent advice on this area.

Income Support is a cash benefit to help people who do not have enough money to live on and who are not working 16 hours a week or more. It can be paid to top up other benefits, or earnings from part-time work, or if you have no money at all. Contact your local social security office or post office for further information.

Department of Social Security's Benefit Agency

Disability Living Allowance is a tax-free benefit paid out regardless of income for people under 65 who have an illness or disability and need help with personal care and getting around. For more information get the leaflet, *Disability Living Allowance*, available from social security offices and post offices.

Department of Social Security's Benefit Agency

Attendance Allowance is a cash benefit for people disabled at or after the age of 65 who need a lot of looking after because of their physical or mental disablement. There are two rates – a lower one for people who need a lot of looking after by day or night, and a higher one for people who need a lot of looking after day and night. It is paid regardless of income and savings and can be paid on top of other benefits, including Income Support. See the leaflet *Attendance Allowance*.

Department of Social Security's Benefit Agency

Disability Working Allowance is paid to people who are able to do some work but have a disability which puts them at a disadvantage in getting a job. It is a tax-free, income related benefit for people who are working for at least 16 hours a week or more. For more details get claim pack *Disabled Persons Tax Credit DPTC/BK1* from your social security office or post office.

Department of Social Security's Benefit Agency

Invalid Care Allowance is a taxable benefit paid to people under the age of 65 who are caring for a severely disabled person for at least 35 hours a week. The carer must be earning no more than £10 a week and the person in their care must be getting the middle or higher rate of Disability Living Allowance or Constant Attendance Allowance. For more information get DS 700, *Invalid Care Allowance claim pack*, from your social security office or post office.	Department of Social Security's Benefit Agency
It is sometimes possible to draw up a **Deed of Covenant**. This is a tax-free means of paying money from one person to another.	You should seek advice on drawing up a Deed of Covenant from a solicitor or accountant
Home Responsibilities Protection is a way of ensuring that people don't get less state pension because they take time off work to stay at home to look after someone who is sick or disabled. The carer must be caring for at least 35 hours a week. For more information get CF 411, *Application form for Home Responsibilities Protection.*	Department of Social Security's Benefit Agency
Council Tax. If the degree of disability is severe, people with Alzheimer's may be exempt from the tax. There is also Council Tax Benefit for those on low incomes. For more information, get Information Sheet 8 on Council Tax from Help the Aged (see p. 77).	Your local council office
Housing Benefit. If you are a tenant you may be able to get help with your rent.	Your local council office

Further information can be found on the website: www.dss.gov.uk

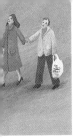

GENERAL GUIDELINES FOR CARING

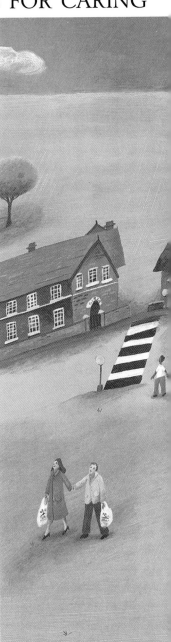

A key to caring for someone with dementia is understanding why they find it increasingly difficult to look after themselves and acknowledging that they may be depressed and anxious at times if they realise what's happening to them.

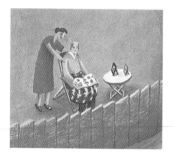

Problems may include:

- They may suffer from loss of memory, a declining power to think, and general confusion. This affects their ability to know *what* they are doing, *why* they are doing it, and *how* to do it. As a result, tasks may be done incorrectly or dangerously, may be left unfinished or not attempted at all.
- They may find it difficult to hold a conversation and express themselves. This leads to an inability to explain their difficulties and to ask for appropriate help.
- They may lose their physical co-ordination. This leads to difficulty and possible risk or danger in carrying out actions.
- They may be embarrassed and frustrated about their declining abilities, and resent having to be helped. This may lead to attempts to conceal their difficulties, resistance to offers of help, and a refusal to carry out certain tasks at all.

KEEP THINGS NORMAL

A diagnosis of dementia does not mean that you must suddenly start treating the person like an invalid. In fact, you should try and make a point of keeping things as normal as possible for as long as possible. Carry on any pursuits which you have both found enjoyable, such as going to the pub, theatre or cinema, listening to music, singing or dancing, unless or until it stops being a pleasure.

Introduce new activities if they seem appropriate –
people with dementia often enjoy the company of
small babies or children, and animals.

RETAIN INDEPENDENCE

There are two major reasons for retaining the person's
ability to carry on independently for as long as
possible. First, it helps them to retain some sense of
dignity and self-respect, and may avoid frustration
being brought on by feeling helpless. Second, it makes
less work for you – the more they can do for
themselves, the less you have to do for them.

Encourage them to carry on with things they can
manage. When something becomes too difficult, don't
give up on it completely – it could be broken down
into smaller or easier bits. But be sure to recognise
when something really is beyond them. Don't show
them up or put them in a position where they fail.
Praise them when they complete a task successfully
or for any help they can give you.

Cut down on what they do on their own slowly and
reluctantly, for as one carer said: 'Once you stop
something, you've only to stop it once and that's it.'

All the same, it is no kindness to the person to expect
them to continue making decisions which are beyond
their capabilities. Brace yourself and start deciding for
yourself what has to be done, when the doctors confirm
that the individual can no longer manage for themselves.

AVOID CONFRONTATION

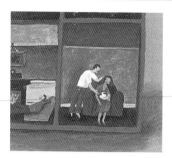

There will be many occasions when you and the person with dementia will have disagreements. You might think it's time they changed their dirty clothes, but they don't agree. They believe someone's stolen money from their purse, you know they haven't. They insist it's perfectly all right to go out shopping dressed in their pyjamas, you'd rather not be with them when they did!

In fact, argument won't usually get you very far. It generally leads only to frustration and aggressive feelings for both of you. It's far better to avoid confrontation whenever you can. Try not to contradict them if they say strange or silly things. Distract their attention if they want to do something inappropriate by changing the subject, or moving them away from the source of the trouble — the chances are that in a moment or two they'll have forgotten what it is they wanted to do anyway.

Experienced carers have lots of suggestions about how to persuade a reluctant patient to do what the carer wants. Avoiding confrontation can be a spur to your imagination.

AVOID CRISES

There will be occasions when the person seems suddenly to get more confused, to behave particularly badly or to cry for no apparent reason and be unable to explain why. These may be caused by crises in their lives – events that seem normal enough to those unaffected by the disease, but alarming to someone who is already confused.

A crisis might be having to hurry to get somewhere on time; meeting too many people at once, even if they are people familiar to them; or going into new and unfamiliar surroundings.

Some of these crises can be easily avoided. Try always to leave plenty of time to prepare for an outing, or to get a task done. Make sure that only one or two friends or relations visit at once. Accompany the patient to new places. If you take them away on holiday, try to go somewhere where both your problems and theirs will be understood. Above all, try and stay calm yourself.

There will be times, though, when crises cannot be avoided, for example, when you are to have a break and a sitter comes in, or the individual is to go to a new day centre. On these occasions simply try to reduce the disorientation they are likely to feel by using a family friend or neighbour as a sitter, or by introducing a stranger in slow stages and with you present. The introduction to a day centre or hospital should also be made gradually.

Don't avoid making any changes at all or stop your social life just to avoid crises for the patient. Sometimes they are inevitable and may be best for them – or for you – in the long run.

ESTABLISH ROUTINES

Routines are vital in caring for someone with dementia. Doing the same thing at the same time every day helps them to remember, and so helps you in your task. And if life is predictable and familiar, there is less chance of increasing confusion.

MAINTAIN A SENSE OF HUMOUR

'The greatest thing I found ... I could get my wife to laugh at everything she did wrong. Everything she did silly, like trying to get her knickers on over her head, I'd say "What are you putting them over there for?" And she'd say: "I'm sure I'm going daft" and we used to laugh.'

There may be times when you can see the lighter side of things, and it is important for your own mental health that you maintain the ability to laugh. The individual too may still be able to enjoy a good joke or a funny situation and it will do you both good to laugh together.

Of course, laughing *with* someone is quite different from laughing *at* them, which no one should ever do.

MAKE THINGS SIMPLER

A person who is already confused will find making straightforward decisions, or carrying out relatively simple tasks, over-complicated and difficult. Taking a bath, for example, involves many separate actions, from putting in the plug to turning on the taps and obtaining the right temperature, getting undressed, and so on.

Try to simplify things: don't offer too many choices (two is probably enough): break tasks down into short, simple sections; if a task becomes too difficult ask them to do only part of it.

Make things simple for yourself too. Don't fight lots of battles at once, but try and solve problems one at a time. That way you stand a better chance of success.

MAKING THINGS SAFER

The dementia patient's difficulties increase the risk of accidents in the home and you should take great care to make your home as safe as possible.

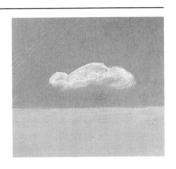

Loss of physical co-ordination increases the likelihood of falls, so you should check your home for danger zones like a loose banister rail, slippery floor mats, awkwardly placed furniture, or carpets which may not have been securely nailed down. You may need to have an extra stair rail fitted, along with handrails in the bath and toilet.

Loss of memory and thinking ability can give rise to risks from a number of everyday activities. A person with dementia may turn on the gas fire but forget to light it; they may drop lighted matches into a waste-paper basket; they may scald themselves on a boiling kettle. Some of the solutions are obvious – switch off the gas at the mains when you go out, don't leave matches around, hide kettle flexes. The list is a long one, and largely a matter of common sense. You should review your home for all potential accidents and take action to avoid them.

MAINTAIN GENERAL FITNESS AND HEALTH

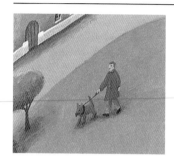

The general state of health of the person with dementia will affect their overall condition. If good general health is maintained it will help to preserve existing physical and mental abilities for as long as possible as well as encouraging independence and sustaining morale. They will need someone to check on their condition, provide a balanced diet and encourage appropriate physical activity.

Keeping a check on the condition of someone with dementia
As the main carer you are the best person to monitor any changes in the patient's condition. They will still suffer from the common colds, coughs and minor complaints that make everyone uncomfortable. However, they are also more prone to certain ailments such as chest infections and more likely to suffer falls. Patients who are unable to move easily and spend much time in one position may develop pressure sores or hypothermia in cold weather (a serious drop in body temperature which can lead to death). All these things need to be carefully watched out for as the person may not be able to explain to you what is wrong and may suffer needlessly. Sometimes you may be able to give a remedy yourself, but do remember that even everyday drugs such as aspirin may worsen their symptoms unless given in small doses. A check with your doctor is advisable if the symptoms are persistent, or if you are unsure what to do.

A district nurse, social worker, or doctor who makes regular home visits can also look out for any changes and reassess the person's needs. They can refer the patient to specialists or services for particular problems such as incontinence. A doctor can prescribe medicines which may give relief from problems such as sleeplessness and wandering at night, depression and delusions, although care needs to be taken when prescribing drugs as they can increase the confusion.

Diet
As the disease progresses there may be problems with the practical side of eating, and tastes for food may alter. But it is most important to try to include all the ingredients of a balanced diet especially as the symptoms of dementia can be worsened by an inadequate diet. Try to provide something the individual likes eating from each of these food groups every day:

- meat, fish, eggs, pulses (dried peas, beans etc)
- fruit and vegetables
- cereals and bread
- dairy produce, milk, cheese etc.

Make sure they drink enough liquid to prevent them becoming dehydrated or constipated. If constipation becomes a problem an increase in high fibre foods such as wholemeal bread, cereals and fruit and vegetables will help. For more dietary advice ask your doctor or health visitor.

Physical activity

Physical activity can be pleasurable as well as helping to preserve existing abilities. The kind of exercise depends on the person's condition and what they are used to but the best kind of activity is usually something they like doing such as walking, dancing, gardening, swimming or playing bowls – at least until these things become impractical. As the disease progresses, a gentle stroll in familiar streets or a park may be more suitable.

KEEP CHANNELS OF COMMUNICATION OPEN

'He can't get the words ... He knows what he wants to say and he expects me to know. He gets angry and very frustrated. The only consolation is that five minutes later he's forgotten and gone on to something else. His frustration doesn't last – it lasts more with us.'

As the person's dementia progresses there will be increasing problems of communication between them and others. There will be difficulties for them in expressing themselves and for carers in explaining things and making themselves understood. This will affect daily activities and the expression of thoughts and feelings.

Talking becomes a problem for the person with dementia. They may use the wrong words, forget words completely, endlessly repeat words or phrases and lose the thread of the conversation. This can be distressing for both them and the carer.

There are several things which can be done to help keep open channels of communication. At a practical level it is extremely important to check that the person's senses are not additionally impaired by, for example, a hearing aid that does not work properly, dentures that are too loose, or glasses that are no longer the correct prescription.

In conversation you should remember to speak clearly, simply and slowly, and to talk about only one topic at a time. Allow extra time for the person to reply. You may need to repeat things several times, find a simpler way of saying something, or guess the sense of what they are saying. If the person is confused remind them of basic information gently, perhaps by using a picture or object. Try not to contradict or embarrass the person by correcting them bluntly.

And, of course, speech is not the only nor the most important way of communicating. Body language – the way we look at a person, how close we move towards them, how we touch them – can be more important than words alone. In the later stages of dementia, looking and touching may be the main ways of expressing affection and care for the person, and their body language gives you clues as to what they mean and how they are feeling as well.

This woman's mother no longer recognises her, but they still communicate:

'I spend an hour sitting with her with my arm round her cuddling her and I tell her that she's the loveliest mother I've ever had, and she just keeps rubbing my hand and face and saying "I like you".'

USE MEMORY AIDS

In the early stages of dementia memory aids may be useful. These are things which may help to jog the memory, clear confusion and disorientation, and keep things as normal as possible.

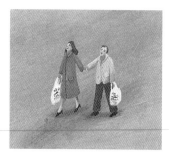

Here are some things carers have found useful:

- frequently remind the individual of the time, day and where they are
- keep a clock with a large clear dial on view
- keep a calendar that can be changed by the day, month and year
- label the doors of rooms such as the bedroom and lavatory with words, pictures and colours
- keep photos of familiar people and the family on view
- leave the individual's personal possessions where they can easily find them
- keep furniture in the same place
- keep checklists of things to do that day, or lists of expected visitors, which can be ticked off
- set things out in the order in which they have to be done
- leave out only the things required, for example, one day's drug supply
- leave a simple clear note with an address if you are going out
- don't forget textures, tastes and smells can also evoke memories

'Their world stands still. He doesn't know what 3.30 or Tuesday mean, so what's the point in telling him?'

'Supposing he remembers? There he is sitting in a wheelchair, can't walk half a yard, and there am I trying to bring his memory back.'

Eventually, however, as the disease progresses, even these aids may become less useful as these comments (see left) from carers show.

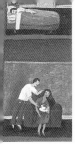

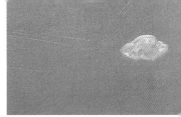

DEALING WITH COMMON PROBLEMS

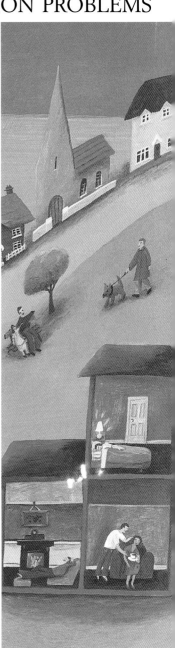

People with dementia may not be able to carry out everyday tasks on their own. For example they may lose their ability to cook or wash themselves, and may not recognise the need to go to the toilet. This chapter highlights common problems and suggests practical solutions on how to deal with them.

DRESSING

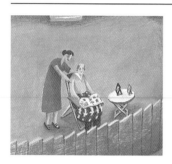

People with dementia don't remember which clothes should be put on, in which order, nor how to put them on. They may end up wearing several skirts and no underwear, or with things on back-to-front or done up incorrectly. They have difficulty doing up buckles, laces, bras and so on. They may not recognise the need to change their clothes, for example, when they are dirty or if they are going to bed. They may choose to wear inappropriate clothing – for example, going out in the daytime in their nightwear.

Possible solutions
Try laying out clothes in the order they have to be put on. Avoid clothes with complicated openings and fastenings. Replace buttons with zips and velcro (but show them how to use them), buckles and belts with elastic, lace-up shoes with slip-ons and men's 'Y' front pants with boxer shorts. Choose women's bras with a front opening.

You may need more persuasive tactics to overcome the last two problems. They may resent interference. Don't argue, try to encourage instead. Set out the clean clothes saying, 'These are the clothes *you* chose to put on', or 'That dress really suits you'. You may have to become tolerant of their preferences. One carer's father frequently wore four pairs of trousers at one time, another's mother went to the day centre in her dressing-gown. But ask yourself if these sorts of things really matter – for whom is 'problem' behaviour a problem?

WASHING AND BATHING

Forgetting to wash and no longer recognising the need may be problems for people with dementia. They may have forgotten what to do, or be unable to wash certain parts of their body because of physical impairment. Some will be unable to climb in or out of the bath safely or manipulate taps. They may be embarrassed by helpers seeing parts of their body usually kept private, and may refuse to wash at all. These problems are increased if they are incontinent and need to wash frequently.

Possible solutions

Try to establish or maintain a routine for washing. You will need much tact. You cannot tell them to wash but perhaps you can emphasise the more pleasant aspects, the comfort of warm water, perfumed soaps and so on. You may have to tell them step by step what to do, wash with them, or clean your own teeth to demonstrate. You may have to help or supervise them because of physical difficulty and risk of accident or injury. There will be difficulties for the carer too if the individual is large or heavy and you need to lift them. You may be able to get a bath attendant or aids such as rails and a bath seat which may alleviate some problems (see *Practical help* on p.38).

Incontinence can be a real problem, especially if embarrassment leads to concealment. And of course it's a problem for the carer who may be just as uncomfortable. Try to be matter-of-fact: 'You know and I know that you're wet, and you'll get sore if you don't wash'. Telling them off or showing that you are upset won't help.

GOING TO THE TOILET

People with dementia may forget to go, leading to incontinence and constipation. They may forget where the toilet is, even in their own home. There may be problems undoing their clothing in time. At night they may lose their way in the dark or mistake some other object such as a waste-bin for the lavatory.

Possible solutions

At regular intervals either remind them or take them. Label the door, or paint it brightly. Make sure clothing can be easily removed. (Try some of the possible solutions from *Dressing* on p.54). Take them before they go to bed. Leave on a lamp with a low wattage bulb, use night-light plugs or stick luminous tape on the wall as a guide. A pot by the side of the bed may help – this used to be common practice for most people when lavatories were outdoors.

COOKING

The problems are most severe if the person with dementia lives alone. The ability to cook even simple meals may be lost. Just buying food and keeping it fresh may be beyond their capacity. They may eat food that has gone bad, or even in some cases, pet food. The gas cooker may be switched on and left unlit, pots may be left to burn. Poor physical co-ordination can lead to burns and scalds or cuts from utensils. The combination of these problems leads to malnourishment in many people with dementia who live alone.

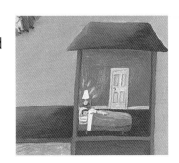

For those living with others, the problems are diminished if the carer cooks for them – the problem then may be for the carer who is unused to buying or cooking food.

Possible solutions

There are safety devices which can be fitted to cookers to prevent some of these problems (see *Practical help* on p.38). Invest in an electric kettle that switches itself off. Remove sharp knives and other potentially dangerous utensils. You may need to visit daily to help or supervise – or arrange for someone else to be there. Try to get the meals-on-wheels service to call (see *Practical help* on p.38), but check to see that the patient knows how to open the container. You may need to put the food out on a plate for them if they don't understand what the carton is for.

Most libraries stock books about cooking on a range of themes – 'for beginners', 'for small households', 'for those on a budget' and so on.

EATING

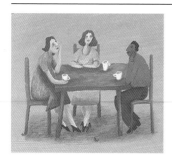

Many people with dementia forget whether or not they have eaten. Some don't want to eat and claim they have just done so, others want to start on the next meal as soon as they have finished the previous one. They may develop strong dislikes of certain foods and cravings for others. Some don't know how to eat. They may forget how to use cutlery and be generally very messy. They may play with their food, not realising it is to go in their mouth. They may be confused by different foods on one plate. Others have physical problems; they can't chew properly and have difficulty swallowing, which could lead to choking. Some forget to drink and may become dehydrated.

Possible solutions
Have regular times for eating, and eat with the person. If the person often wants to start another meal soon after the last one, keep some washing up in the sink to show the remains of the last meal. If they will eat only certain foods you may have to ask your doctor about diet and vitamin supplements.

Don't worry about table manners – spoons are easier than knives and forks, and fingers came first of all! Use plastic tablecloths and place mats so mess can be easily cleaned up.

You may have to remind them how to eat by talking them through each stage, or show them by eating something yourself. Sometimes spoonfeeding may be necessary. Try to keep food simple. Cut it up small or keep it to one texture – soft, thick foods are best. A mixture of liquid and solid may lead them to swallow instead of chewing and could result in choking. Check that dentures fit and are left clean.

Make sure that the person has several drinks a day and that the drinks are not too hot – they may have lost their judgement. You may need to use a spillproof cup like the ones sold for children.

GOING OUT ALONE AND SHOPPING

The most worrying problem for many carers is the patient's safety (see also the section on *Wandering* on p.62). Traffic presents a threat on even the quietest roads and crowded, busy streets or shopping centres can confuse and alarm. The patient may not recognise even familiar places, and become lost and frightened. Other people are not always helpful and may interpret confused behaviour as drunkenness.

If a person with dementia is shopping for themself there are additional problems of remembering what they went out to buy and handling money.

Possible solutions

Many carers are rightly reluctant to prevent the patient going out alone as it is often the last thing they can do on their own. Encourage the person to walk in a park or other area safe from traffic and crowds. If this is not possible you may have to accompany them – perhaps take them part of the way to a point where they cannot go wrong, or meet them on the return journey. One carer relied on a well-trained and trusted dog to help her husband cross the road and bring him home.

Persuade them to carry identification – a bracelet or card explaining that they might become confused and showing where you can be contacted. Or sew a name tape into a pocket.

If they are shopping give them a clear note and only the amount of money they will need. They will be able to buy only one or two straightforward items. If they need clothes you will have to go with them. Do not be embarrassed to explain the problem to shop assistants who are usually most helpful once they understand.

DRIVING

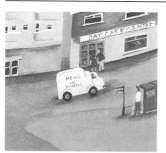

People with dementia are able to continue driving in the early stages of the disease. However, the DVLA should be told that the person is suffering from dementia so that regular checks on their ability to drive can be made.

Possible solutions

Once you feel that someone should stop driving, broach the subject with them gently. Some may be pleased to be rid of the responsibility driving brings. Others, who resent their loss of independence, may find giving up driving particularly hard. If gentle persuasion doesn't dissuade them from driving, you will have to take firmer action. In the first instance, offer to drive yourself (if you can), or suggest using public transport. If need be, hide the car keys or immobilise the car (go to a garage for advice about the easiest way to do this). Remember, many insurance companies require a medical certificate of fitness before insuring older drivers.

ALCOHOL AND CIGARETTES

If the patient is in the habit of drinking alcohol in moderation, there is no reason why it should be stopped. Having a drink may be one of their remaining pleasures, and something you can enjoy together. You should take care, however, that alcohol is not left out where they can help themselves. If they are on medication, remember to check with the doctor or pharmacist that the drugs mix safely with alcohol.

The use of cigarettes represents a greater danger. People with dementia are not safe with matches, and they may smoke in bed, leave lighted cigarettes on the edge of armchairs, or throw them away in waste-paper baskets.

Possible solutions
Give the patient a cigarette lighter which cuts off when their finger is removed from the ignition button. If they really need to smoke, it should be only under

strict supervision. It is far better to dissuade them from smoking. If persuasion fails, choose a moment when they are otherwise occupied to remove their cigarettes. It may be reassuring to know that many people with dementia forget to smoke so don't miss the habit once it is broken.

WANDERING

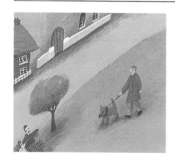

Wandering is a common and difficult problem to deal with. People with dementia may wander aimlessly or anxiously around the home, or wander around the neighbourhood having slipped secretly out of the house. They may wander long distances to old haunts and get lost. You will be worried about their safety and their own bewilderment or fear.

Possible solutions

If you can work out a reason for the wandering you may find a solution. Sometimes wandering results from general restlessness and boredom and is a sign that the person needs more stimulation or physical activity. They may be searching for things they think are lost. Keeping personal possessions on view may help here (see also *Losing things and accusations of theft* on p.66). Often they feel insecure and may need both the emotional reassurance that you care and the concrete reassurance of things being kept in the same places and routines maintained. Wandering frequently starts after a visit to a strange place – after a holiday, for example – or after a change of habit – such as starting at a day centre, in which case it may help if you go with them a few times until the change becomes familiar. Moving home can be very distressing for people with dementia and should be avoided if at all possible.

If you can find no apparent reason then you have to prevent them wandering where they will be at risk. You may have to lock some rooms at home, or fix up a stair gate – like the ones sold to restrain children, but check that they cannot climb over it. You'll need to install unfamiliar or difficult locks on street doors. Put the locks on the bottom of the door where they are less likely to find them.

An identity bracelet worn by the patient giving details of how you can be contacted is an additional safety measure. If they do still manage to wander off, contact the police who will then keep a look out too.

NIGHT DISTURBANCE

Many people with dementia are restless at night and disturb the whole household by wandering and making a noise. This can be one of the most wearying problems for carers.

Possible solutions

Again, if you can find a reason you might be able to alleviate the problem. Some of the more obvious reasons may be that the person:

- is looking for the toilet
- sleeps too much in the daytime

- goes to bed too early
- needs less sleep
- is not comfortable
- wakes up and is confused or frightened
- thinks it is daytime.

Make sure they have been to the toilet before going to bed (see also *Going to the toilet* on p.56 and *Incontinence* on p.66). Try to discourage long sleeps during the day, perhaps by increasing physical activity. Try to make them as comfortable as possible. A bedside lamp with a low-wattage bulb left on may help if the person wakes up frightened. Sometimes talking gently to the person will reassure them too and send them back to sleep. If they think it's daytime or they think they need to get up for some reason you might have to play along with them as arguing could lead to upset. One carer spoke of her husband who regularly woke at night wanting to go to the shops. She always said, 'All right then, let's go,' walked him round the room and back to bed by which time he'd forgotten where he was going.

If nothing seems to work and the disruption to your own sleep makes you unable to cope, you will have to ask your doctor about medication.

REPETITIVE QUESTIONING AND ACTIONS

This can be extremely irritating for carers! Usually the individual is unaware of what they're doing, although their behaviour may reflect underlying anxiety or insecurity.

Possible solutions

There's no point getting angry or saying, 'I've just told you ten times.' Try to distract them by talking about something else or giving them a different activity. Sometimes writing down the answer helps. Reassuring them of your concern may reduce insecurity. You may also have to develop your skills at turning a deaf ear.

CLINGING

Some people with dementia become reluctant to let their carer out of their sight and follow them from room to room. This can be very distressing for you, as it means you're allowed no privacy, often even to go to the lavatory.

They probably behave like this because they're feeling insecure, and the care-giver represents security. When they see you leave the room, they forget that you will come back and get frightened.

Possible solutions

While you're gone, give them some simple task to do or use the clock to point out when you'll return. Reassure them that you'll be back when the task is finished or when the clock reads a certain time.

If this happens to you, it is important that you use sitters or find some other way of getting a break.

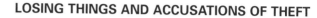

LOSING THINGS AND ACCUSATIONS OF THEFT

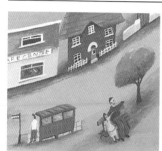

Many people with dementia really do forget where they have put things; others deliberately hide things and then forget. In either case they may accuse you or someone else of stealing the missing items.

Possible solutions
Try not to take their accusations too seriously. Don't deny the charge and get into an argument – it won't be possible to reason with them and they will become more upset. Try to find out if they have a regular hiding place such as under the mattress or in an old shoe. Keep replacements of essential items such as keys or glasses. Put away or lock up valuables, money or dangerous things. Get into the habit of checking rubbish bins before emptying them. Make sure that other people who help care for the person are aware of the problem.

INCONTINENCE

Many people with dementia may be occasionally incontinent and wet the bed. Regular bladder incontinence and bowel incontinence is less usual. But even the occasional accident can be difficult to deal with. It is embarrassing and degrading for them and distasteful for the carer who has to clean up.

However, incontinence is a condition that can be greatly improved by medical treatment, so ask your doctor or health visitor for help.

66

If incontinence becomes frequent or develops suddenly always check with your doctor, as there could be a medical reason.

There could be several reasons for occasional incontinence:

- they forget to go
- they can't get to the toilet in time
- they can't undo their clothing easily
- they can't find their way at night
- they have an attack of diarrhoea.

Possible solutions
- Take the person to the toilet regularly.
- If the toilet is upstairs or some distance from where they spend most of their time try to get a commode (see *Practical help* on p.38).
- Clothing can be adapted by using velcro instead of buttons or zips. Men's 'Y' front pants can be replaced by boxer shorts. Your district nurse can tell you about the special clothing that is available. If you're not already in touch with your district nurse ask your doctor to put you in touch.
- Provide a pot for night-time use. Use luminous tapes to mark the route to the toilet. Always take them before they go to bed and if it prevents a wet bed take them during the night.
- Keep a check on their diet. If they are not eating enough roughage they may develop constipation which can lead to a blocked bowel and leaking

diarrhoea. Increase vegetables, fruits and whole-grain cereals.

- Try to reduce embarrassment by adopting a matter-of-fact approach, directing their attention to the task of cleaning and washing and avoiding any recriminations.

- To protect your furniture use washable covers over dustbin liners. Beds can be protected by using a plastic sheet between a draw sheet (a sheet folded in half and tucked in across the bed).

- Special pads and pants are available from chemist shops or through health authorities (ask your district nurse). Some local authorities provide a laundry service (see *Practical help* on p.38).

DELUSIONS AND HALLUCINATIONS

Delusions are ideas that are imaginary, but that seem very real to the person experiencing them. Someone suffering from delusions may believe that there are some people who want to kill or harm them, or that objects which are simply mislaid or hidden have been stolen, even by members of the family.

Someone suffering hallucinations sees or hears things that aren't actually there. They may wake to see figures at the foot of the bed, or hear dead relatives talking to them.

Possible solutions

Both delusions and hallucinations are imaginary, but they can give rise to genuine feelings of anxiety or panic, and should be taken seriously.

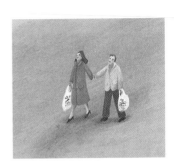

When the patient is experiencing a delusion or hallucination, don't argue with them or tell them they are mistaken. Remember they are outside the person's control so becoming angry or impatient with them will not help. If the delusion concerns a missing object, for example, try to find it, rather than deny it has been stolen. If the person is distressed by a hallucination explain that you understand what they are feeling, but also that other people cannot see or hear what frightens them. Try to comfort them, perhaps by putting an arm round them or holding their hand, and try to distract their attention on to something real around them.

If the person you are caring for begins to suffer from distressing delusions or hallucinations, you should see your doctor. It could be that medication is causing the problem, or the problem might itself respond to drugs.

SEXUAL RELATIONSHIPS

The sexual relationship in a marriage is very private and personal and not something that many carers can talk about easily. While dementia does not necessarily affect sexual relationships, the patient's attitude to lovemaking may alter. They may not respond to affectionate gestures that you make or they may lose interest altogether. They may simply forget about it.

You may find that you lose interest yourself because of the stresses and tiredness brought on by caring for your loved-one. You may find it difficult to make love with a person whose personality has changed so much.

Occasionally, a person with dementia may become more demanding.

Possible solutions
There is no simple solution to a complex and sensitive issue such as this. If you find that your sexual relationship is becoming a problem, you should try and talk to an understanding person about it. There are counsellors trained to talk to people about such problems. Your doctor should be able to put you in touch with someone.

INAPPROPRIATE SEXUAL BEHAVIOUR

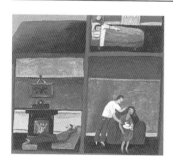

In some cases a person suffering from dementia may exhibit inappropriate sexual behaviour, such as undressing in public, exposing themselves, or aimlessly fondling their genitals. In fact, such behaviour is unlikely to be sexual at all. Appearing naked in the sitting-room may simply be the result of forgetting they should get dressed, or of losing their way to the bathroom. A man found 'exposing' himself, may only be trying to urinate in an unsuitable place. One carer's mother seen 'exposing' herself in the street, had wandered out in the cold in her nightdress and pulled it up around her shoulders to try and keep warm.

Possible solutions

Behaviours such as these can cause severe embarrassment to carers, but your understanding of the problem – and explaining it to others – should lessen your embarrassment. If the patient touches their genitals in public, don't make a scene, but try to discourage them gently. If they appear naked, or start undressing themselves, remove them calmly to another room. It may be worth checking that clothing is not uncomfortably tight, or fastenings broken. In those rare cases where people complain and police or other officials become involved a truthful explanation usually receives a sympathetic response. Whatever happens, do not worry that this kind of sexual action will lead to harmful sexual behaviour – it won't.

VIOLENCE AND AGGRESSION

The patient's frustration or over-reaction to a difficult situation may occasionally erupt into aggression and violence. When it is directed at the carer it is especially distressing.

The person may also show anger or aggression towards other family members. Several carers mentioned a particular problem with teenage children, whom people with dementia often seem to resent, perhaps because they represent a youthfulness and hope which they know is past for them.

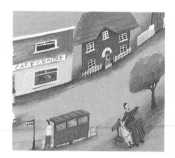

Possible solutions

Whatever you do, do not respond to aggression with aggression. It will only make matters worse. Instead, stay calm yourself – count to 100 if need be – and try to distract their attention. Find out what brings on the reaction – frustration at a difficult task, a certain person's presence, rushing to be ready on time – and try to avoid it in future.

If episodes of violence and aggression become frequent, you should talk to your doctor about medication which may help.

FAILURE TO RECOGNISE PEOPLE

A person with dementia often lives in the past. If a man thinks of himself as still in his forties, it is not surprising that he denies he is married to someone in her sixties or seventies or that he thinks his 40-year-old daughter is his wife.

Possible solutions

Keeping out large photographs of family occasions through the years, so that the person with dementia sees that he (or she) has also grown older has helped some families. Understanding what is happening can relieve the distress carers feel at rejection.

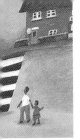

LEGAL MATTERS

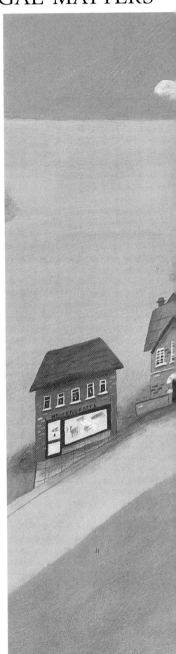

As the dementia progresses, the person with dementia may no longer be able to handle their own financial and other affairs. But help is available from a range of professionals and services. This chapter explains some legal matters and refers you to sources of information.

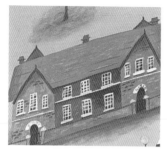

On a day-to-day level, this may not cause any problems. It is relatively easy for you to take over the regular and routine tasks such as paying bills, collecting the person's pension, paying the rent and so on. You can get a form from the DSS which allows you to collect their pension or benefits. It is important to obtain advice about Enduring Power of Attorney and the Court of Protection at the earliest possible stage (see below). Understanding bank managers and others who may require the patient's signature on documents may allow you to sign on their behalf. It would be a good idea to get a joint bank account if you have not already got one.

However, it is not wise to allow the situation to drift along. If the patient's affairs are at all complicated – if they own a business or property, for example – it is important that you should get expert legal advice as soon as possible about any problems that may arise, before they arise. For example, spouses who own their home jointly may find that they are unable to sell it, or if they do, that they are not entitled to all the proceeds of the sale.

English law provides two ways for a person's affairs to be taken over. The first is Enduring Power of Attorney. The second is the Court of Protection.

Enduring Power of Attorney

This gives one person the legal right to manage another person's affairs. It can only be given when the person creating the Enduring Power of Attorney is deemed mentally capable. The Enduring Power of Attorney Act 1985, makes it possible to appoint an attorney who has the power to act after the person becomes mentally incapable. The person still has to be mentally capable when creating this power, so it may become common practice for people to appoint an attorney when making their will, in case they should ever become mentally incapable.

The Court of Protection
This court can appoint a Receiver – a member of the family, a solicitor or the Receivership Division of the Public Trust Office – to take over a person's financial affairs if that person has become mentally incapable. This is a costly and long drawn out process and is only worth doing if there is a lot of money involved or the person's finances are very complicated. For these reasons the Enduring Power of Attorney is nearly always preferable to other forms of receivership/guardianship etc. However, the Public Trust Office point out that someone can be authorised to deal with a person's property and finances under a Short Procedure Order where the assets are limited.

You should go to your nearest Citizens' Advice Bureau, Neighbourhood Law Centre or family solicitor for advice on any of these matters.

USEFUL ORGANISATIONS

Some of these organisations publish their own material on dementia and caring for people at home. Some run groups for carers. These are national organisations and many can provide details of local groups.

AGE CONCERN ENGLAND
Astral House
1268 London Road
London SW16 4ER
Information Line:
0800 00 99 66
www.ace.org.uk

AGE CONCERN SCOTLAND
113 Rose Street
Edinburgh EH2 3DT
Phone: 0131 220 3345

AGE CONCERN NORTHERN IRELAND
3 Lower Crescent
Belfast BT7 1NR
Phone: 028 9024 5729

AGE CONCERN CYMRU
4th Floor
1 Cathedral Road
Cardiff CF11 9SD
Phone: 029 2037 1566

ALZHEIMER'S SOCIETY
Gordon House
10 Greencoat Place
London SW1P 1PH
Phone: 020 7306 0606
Helpline: 0845 300 0336
www.alzheimers.org.uk

ALZHEIMER'S SCOTLAND
Action on Dementia
22 Drumsheugh Gardens
Edinburgh EH3 7RN
Phone: 0131 243 1453
Dementia Helpline:
0808 808 3000

CROSSROADS – CARING FOR CARERS
10 Regent Place
Rugby
Warwickshire CV21 2PN
Phone: 01788 573 653

CARERS NATIONAL ASSOCIATION
20 – 25 Glasshouse Yard
London EC1A 4JT
Phone: 020 7490 8818
Carers Line:
0808 808 7777
www.carersnorth.demon.co.uk

CITIZENS ADVICE BUREAU
see your local telephone directory (if you can't find the address of CAB in your local telephone directory contact the National Association of Citizens Advice Bureaux who will tell you where your nearest office is).

COUNSEL AND CARE
Twyman House
16 Bonny Street
London NW1 9PG
Phone: 020 7241 8555
Advice on residential care and benefits:
0845 300 7585
www.counselandcare.org.uk
email:
advice@counselandcare.org.uk

DISABLED LIVING FOUNDATION
380 – 384 Harrow Road
London W9 2HU
Phone: 020 7289 6111
Helpline: 0845 130 9177
www.dlf.org.uk

ELDERLY ACCOMMODATION COUNSEL
3rd floor, 89 Albert Embankment
London SE1 7TP
Phone: 020 7820 1343
www.housingcare.org

HEALTH EDUCATION BOARD FOR SCOTLAND
Woodburn House
Canaan Lane
Edinburgh EH10 4SG
Phone: 0131 536 5500
www.hebs.scot.nhs.uk

HEALTH PROMOTION DIVISION, NATIONAL ASSEMBLY FOR WALES
Ffynnon-las
Tŷ Glas Avenue
Llanishen
Cardiff CF14 5EZ
Phone: 029 2075 2222
www.hpw.wales.gov.uk

HELP THE AGED
207 – 221 Pentonville Road
London N1 9UZ
Phone: 020 7278 1114
SeniorLine: 0808 800 6565
www.helptheaged.org.uk

MIND (NATIONAL ASSOCIATION FOR MENTAL HEALTH)
Granta House
15 – 19 Broadway
London E15 4BQ
Phone: 020 8519 2122
Infoline: 08457 660 163
Publications:
020 8221 9666
www.mind.org.uk

NATIONAL ASSOCIATION OF CITIZENS ADVICE BUREAUX
Myddleton House
115 – 123 Pentonville Road
London N1 9LZ
Phone: 020 7833 2181
www.nacab.org.uk

PRINCESS ROYAL TRUST FOR CARERS
142 Minories
London EC3N 1LB
Phone: 020 7480 7788
www.carers.org
email: info@carers.org

All the leaflets mentioned on pp.39–40 are free and can be obtained by writing to your local Social Security (Benefit Agency) office

LOCAL INFORMATION

NAMES, TELEPHONE NUMBERS AND ADDRESSES FOR EASY REFERENCE

YOUR DOCTOR

DISTRICT NURSE

HEALTH VISITOR

HOSPITAL SERVICES

LOCAL AUTHORITY SOCIAL WORKER

MEALS-ON-WHEELS

HOME HELPS

VOLUNTARY ORGANISATIONS

LOCAL CARERS' GROUP

OPTICIAN

DENTIST

CHIROPODIST

OTHER